Essential Oils Guide Book

The Complete Reference Guide to Essential Oil

Remedies, Recipes, History, Uses, Safety, and How

to Choose the Best Essential Oils

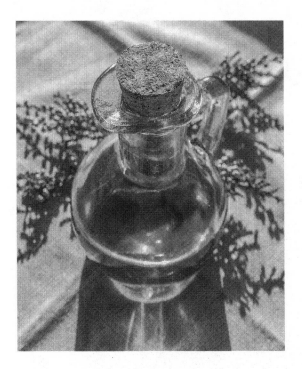

Essential Oils Guide Book

The Complete Reference Guide to Essential Oil Remedies, Recipes, History, Uses, Safety, and How to Choose the Best Essential Oils

Copyright © 2018 Olivia Banks

Published by CAC Publishing LLC.

ISBN 978-1-948489-88-1 paperback

ISBN 978-1-948489-87-4 eBook

Contents

Introduction

Think about the beautiful fragrance of your favorite flower. Maybe it is a rose. Maybe it's jasmine. Perhaps you have a favorite herb that you cook with, like oregano or rosemary, that evokes that wonderful aroma. All of these luscious scents come from the plant's essential oils.

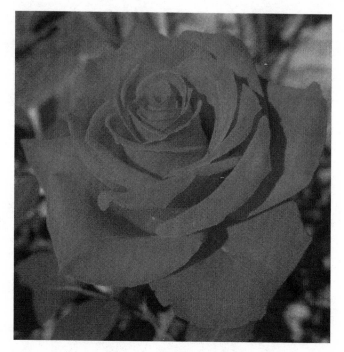

Photo by Hamachidori

What Are Essential Oils?

All plants have oils that are essential to the plant's function. These oils are called "essential" because they provide essential functions and protections for the plant. These oils are extracted from the plant and bottled in a pure and highly concentrated form for all sorts of uses. The oils can be extracted from leaves and other parts of the plants by crushing or distilling to release the essential oils.

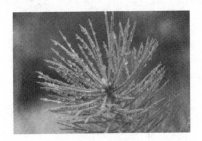

Essential oils are not really oils at all, because they don't consist of the fatty acids that make an oil an oil as we know it. They are highly concentrated plant extracts that many people consider to be the soul or life force of the plant.

How Essential Oils Help Plants

We can all take a lesson from plants and how they use essential oils and extrapolate it for our own use. Think of essential oils as a plant's active chemical compounds that serve as a built-in natural protection against the environment. The citronella plant is a great example. Have you ever used a citronella candle on your patio to ward off mosquitoes? If so, that candle is using the natural essential oil in the citronella plant to keep pests at bay.

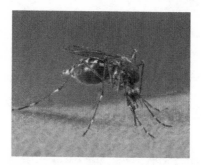

Photo courtesy of US Department of Agriculture

Plants have oils that provide protection and healing for the plant itself. Each plant has different oils which translate to a distinctive smell for each plant. That's why roses and rosemary don't smell the same (thank goodness!) Some oils attract insects to the plant in order to pollinate it, like roses, jasmine, citrus blooms and other sweet-smelling flowers. Other oils are sharp and pungent, like citronella, telling pests to stay away.

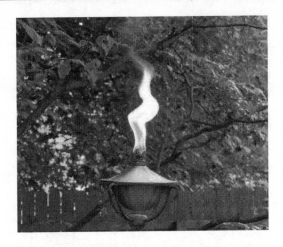

Each oil is unique with its own microscopic building blocks called volatile aromatic compounds (VAC) that determine the oils' unique properties. These compounds are termed "volatile" because they very quickly change state from one form to another—in this case from liquid to gas. When you first open a bottle, the strong aroma comes from the oil changing into a gaseous state.

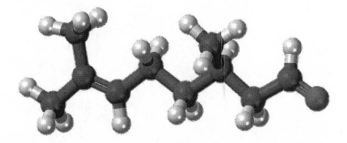

Amazingly, more than 3,000 plant VACs have been discovered by scientists worldwide. Interestingly, slightly different species of the same plant all have slightly different VACs. Oil compositions of the same species can vary depending on where the plant is grown, and climate conditions like geography, altitude, temperature and humidity.

How Essential Oils Help Humans

Essential oils work for plants, so why wouldn't they work for humans? The essential oil VAC building blocks are molecules small enough to penetrate your cells. Essential oils differ from other oils like fatty vegetable oils which are larger molecules too large to penetrate cells. Therefore, they can be used for cooking, but not for therapeutic health benefit.

All of the protective, healing qualities that the plants possess in their stems, bark, roots, leaves and flowers have been harnessed and bottled into the essential oils we humans use today.

The Market For Essential Oils

The harnessing and bottling market is a huge global market. Indeed, a new report by Grand View Research shows that the global market for essential oils will reach nearly $14 billion in just a few years, by 2024. Essential oils have exploded onto the scene as more and more people seek natural remedies and organic products. Today, people all over the world use essential oils for a wide range of physical and emotional applications. Oils are used as single oils or can be mixed with other oils to create powerful and complex essential oil blends.

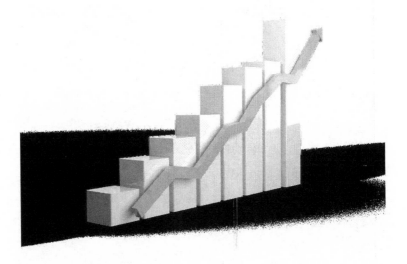

History of Essential Oils

In today's modern world, we have so many synthetic products. More and more, people are shying away from synthetics and opting for more natural products like the essential oils. Ancient people didn't have synthetics and had to naturally rely on botanicals. The modern essential oil market represents the evolution of thousands of years of essential oils use. Indeed, many modern pharmaceuticals are derived from plants. Let's explore the history, shall we?

The ancient world was heavily intermingled with the plant world. They used plant extracts for religion, medicine, food preparation and beauty.

Egypt

The earliest written and recorded uses of essential oils were in Egypt, where plant life flourished thanks to the very fertile Nile River valley. Historical records show that Egypt had an abundance of food and a booming agricultural industry. The Egyptian civilization was progressive in many ways, including urban planning, government, and most of all medicine.

Historians reference the 1500 B.C. Ebers Papyrus as one of the earliest known medical texts from Egypt. It is believed to have been a copy from earlier texts dating back to 3000 B.C. The scroll contains rituals for medical ceremonies, recipes, and uses of botanicals for all kinds of things, including mummification.

Of course, Egypt wrote the book (literally) on how to mummify bodies in preparation for burial, and this early text references use of juniper, cedar and cinnamon oils in preparing the bodies.

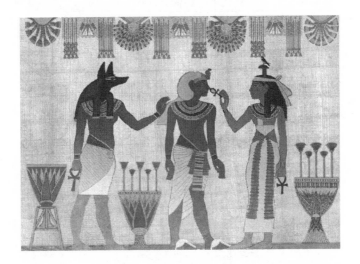

Egyptians used oils not just for mummification, but also in many aspects of everyday life, in many religious ceremonies and herbal remedies for medical purposes. The Egyptian culture had a focus on beauty, and many plant oils were used to concoct beauty treatments. The famous Egyptian queen Cleopatra was given a wonderful gift by her love Marc Antony—he gave her a spa near the Dead Sea. Clearly Antony is a man after every girl's heart, and Cleopatra regularly used the spa's natural resources like salt, clay, and essential oils to maintain her legendary beauty.

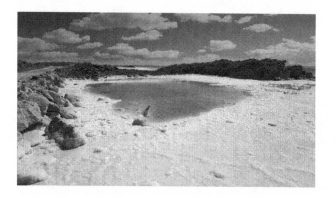

Egypt's ruling pharaoh families wore expensive perfumes made from essential oils, and temple priests used many oils for spiritual ceremonies. These priests also doubled as doctors, so they used many oils to prepare medicines and ointments.

Amazingly, archaeologists have discovered ancient pictorial hieroglyphics on Egyptian temple walls that show essential oils being extracted and used. Plants and their oils were revered in the Egyptian culture. When scientists found King Tutankhamen's tomb in 1922, they discovered over 50 alabaster jars thought to hold essential oils, left there for the pharaoh to use in the afterlife.

Although historians largely give credit to Egypt as the first culture to widely use essential oils, it turns out that ancient China and India were also using these oils around the same time period.

China

In China, plants have been an integral part of medicine for centuries, and continue to be today. The 2700 B.C. text known as Shennong's Herbal is the oldest known Chinese text. It contains details on how the ancient Chinese healers used nearly 400 medicinal plants. Shennong is regarded as the father of Chinese herbal medicine; he was also a ruler who taught the people agriculture. Shennong used himself as a guinea pig and ingested hundreds of herbs and plants to test their effects. He is largely credited as being the discoverer of tea and the inventor of acupuncture. Like Shennong, Huangdi, also called the Yellow Emperor, wrote a book on medicine which detailed the important use of essential oils. Amazingly, Huangdi's book is still used by Chinese medicine practitioners to this day. Indeed, China is the largest producer of essential oils in the world today.

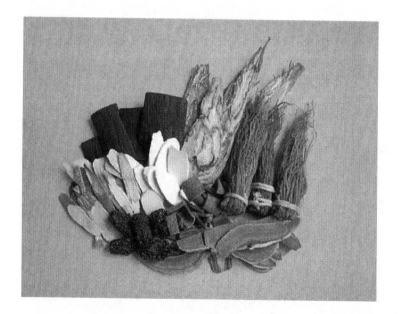

India

Like in China, ancient India used essential oils as a core part of their Ayurvedic practices. Still used today,

Ayurvedic practice is a naturopathic approach to healing that combines practical elements of medicine with spiritual and philosophical beliefs.

Although historians cannot accurately pinpoint a beginning, Ayurvedic medicine is thought to have been practiced for at least 5,000 years. Indeed it is still widely practiced in India, as well as other parts of the world, even today.

One of the principle Ayurvedic practices is aromatherapy and massage. Indian literature, as far back as 2000 B.C., discusses doctors' use of oils like cinnamon, ginger and sandalwood with massage to ease patient symptoms.

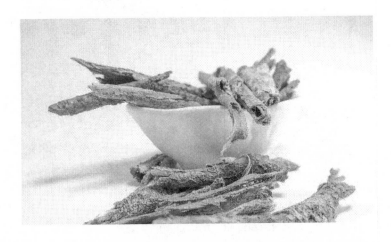

The term "Ayurveda" means "life knowledge", and the Indian sacred text known as the Vedas mentions more than 700 different plants and herbs used for religious and medical purposes. For example, basil is considered a sacred plant of India. It is believed to bestow the properties of energy, love and devotion, and also believed to have the power to open one's heart and mind. Basil is widely accepted in India and used to strengthen compassion, faith and clarity of thought.

Ayurvedic principles have worldwide influence in modern times, thanks to practitioners like Deepak Chopra and other people across the globe who have established training institutions.

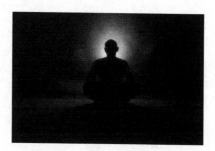

Greeks

The ancient Greeks and Romans derived much of their knowledge from the Egyptians, including use of essential oils. The Greek father of modern medicine,

Hippocrates, kept records of medicinal uses for over 300 plants. He still influences medicine today as doctors still take the Hippocratic oath in his name. Hippocrates often prescribed hot baths with aromatic oils added to the water and massage with essential oils.

During Hippocrates lifetime, a plague hit Athens, and he fumigated the city with essential oils to keep the pestilence from spreading. Today, we know that plague is caused by an infectious bacteria, and we also know that oils, like oregano, have antibacterial properties. Although Hippocrates did not have our modern knowledge, he was obviously on the right track. He always prescribed all kinds of essential oil treatments for wounded soldiers on the battlefields.

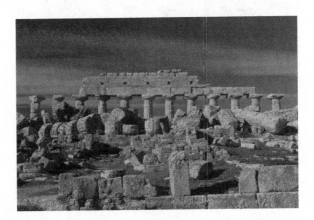

Hippocrates' colleague Theophrastus talked about the "perfumes", meaning essential oils with medicinal properties because of the effects they had on various ailments. He talked of plasters and poultices being used to treat abscesses and tumors as well as internal injuries. Interestingly, the Greeks had already figured out that if these oils are applied externally to the skin, they seep in to repair internal tissues. Indeed, oils are widely used today for this very purpose.

Romans

Like the Greeks, ancient Romans were influenced by Egyptians and the Greeks, particularly in the area of health care. More than any culture before them, Romans used essential oils voluminously. They ate them, they drank them, they bathed in them, they breathed them in, and they had massages using them. The oils were a part of daily life. In particular, the Romans were bath fanatics and known to bathe up to several times a day in waters laced with essential oils. They used oils for hair and body care, and scented their beds with oils like lavender, a practice still widely done today. Romans had master perfumers, who used the most exotic oils to create amazing blends.

Greek physician Dioscorides was employed as an army doctor in Rome, and he wrote a multi-volume book on herbal medicine in 1 A.D. In the book were 600 remedies, many which are still used today. He wrote about juniper berry as a diuretic, marjoram as a sedative, and cypress for treating diarrhea.

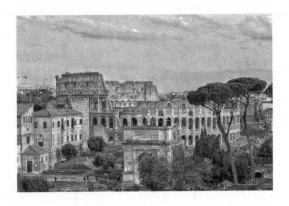

Essential oils are even mentioned in the Christian Bible. Shortly after Christ's birth, the three wise men brought gifts of frankincense and myrrh, two of the oldest essential oils. The Bible has dozens of references to medicinal plants, and mentions at least 12 essential oils, like cinnamon and cedarwood. In the story of Moses's Exodus, the Bible mentions a holy anointing oil containing cassia, clove and olive oils.

Middle Ages – Europe

In the Middle Ages, essential oil use experienced a temporary setback when the Catholic Church denounced many of Hippocrates' teachings, like bathing for healing. Despite the Pope's ruling, many monks kept using plant medicine as cures in their villages, and by the 1600s, herbal medicine was once again widely used. By the 1800s, most of Europe's pharmacies, such as in England, Germany and France, were using and prescribing essential oils for a variety of illnesses.

In France, large flower growers were also using the oils as a commercial business by supplying them to the perfume houses which the French are still known for today. One day, scientists took notice that men who worked at the flower growers were generally healthy, even though disease like tuberculosis were sweeping the rest of France. The curiosity of these early researchers led to the first known laboratory test of anti-bacterial properties of the oils in 1887.

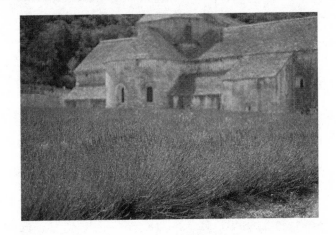

Later, in 1910, a scientific discovery occurred by accident, as so many often do. French chemist Rene-Maurice Gattefosse suffered severe burns to his hands and arms as a result of a laboratory explosion. His hands quickly showed signs of severe blistering so he used the only remedy he had and dipped his hands into a large container of lavender oil. Gattefosse was astonished that one dip stopped the burning.

Gattefosse was a chemist, but wasn't interested in medicine until his personal experience changed his path. He soon began investigating how oils could be used to treat World War I soldiers. Gattefosse is famous for creating the term "aromatherapie". Several decades later, Parisian medical doctor Jean Valnet, followed in Gattefosse's footsteps in another moment of serendipity. He ran out of antibiotics during the Indochina War in the 1950s. Remembering Gattefosse's story, he began using essential oils as antiseptics. Since he was stationed in China, the oils were in ready supply. Valnet credited the oils for saving many soldiers. After the war, he continued his research and even published an authoritative text entitled The Practice of Aromatherapy in 1964. The book is still widely recognized today as the basis for the modern global essential oil movement.

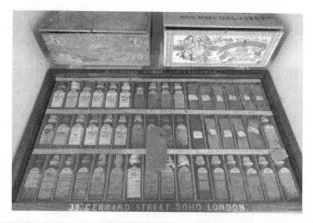

Exhibit in the Tekniska Museet, Stockholm, Sweden

Twenty years later, more French scientists, Daniel Pénoël and Pierre Franchomme, provided clinical uses for over 270 essential oils and published their book L'aromatherapie Exactement in 1990, still used today as the primary reference book for medical benefits of essential oils.

Health Benefits of Essential Oils

Clearly, ancient cultures and modern-day scientists were on to something. What they knew from observation, modern scientists know from research and detailed knowledge of how cells function. Today, we know the exact mechanisms of how essential oils work.

Antibacterial

Scientists have turned to essential oils as an alternative to antibiotics, which bacteria are increasingly becoming resistant to. "The loss of antibiotics due to antimicrobial resistance is potentially one of the most important challenges the medical and animal-health communities will face in the 21st century," says Dr. Cyril Gay, the senior national program leader at the United States Department of Agriculture (USDA).

Some estimates predict that these drug-resistant bacteria will cause more than 10 million deaths in the next 30 years, by 2050.

Livestock consume antibiotics, and then the meat is consumed by humans. The out-of-control use in agriculture has led to the creation of superbugs with dire consequences to humans. The large majority of antibiotics used on livestock are also used to treat human diseases, and that is why the consequences are so dire. The USDA has turned to essential oils research as a potential antibiotic alternative, and some of it has been very promising. An October 2014 study showed that oregano oil fed to chickens greatly reduced the occurrence of a common poultry infection called ascites.

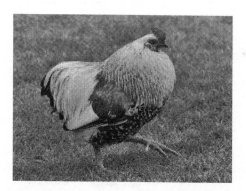

In another study, a feed meal made of oregano, cinnamon and chili peppers suppressed a common intestinal infection and even resulted in the chickens gaining more weight. Another team of researchers used a similar concoction of turmeric, chili pepper, and shiitake mushrooms. The USDA is currently conducting a multi-year study examining the use of several essential oils like citrus oils as antibiotic alternatives.

The USDA and other researchers have compared antibiotics with essential oil use and have found them to be comparable. In one example, rosemary and oregano oils had similar results to the common poultry antibiotic avilamycin. At the University of Georgia, a blend of oils was effective at stopping the spread of salmonella. There is strong evidence that these essential oils are very effective against the intestinal bacteria that often affect livestock.

Human research has shown similar promising results, although the studies are rare and tend to be smaller scale studies. American researchers have studied tea tree oil and its effect on staph infections; wounds treated with the oil healed faster, and lemongrass oil reduced the antibiotic resistant dangerous form of staph called MRSA.

Many scientific labs around the globe are testing all kinds of combinations of essential oils, and consistently, research shows that these oils can fight numerous pathogens, regular and antibiotic-resistant. Even when antibiotics are given, using oils can reduce the amount of drugs a person must take. Basil oil and rosemary oil slowed the growth of 60 strains of *E. coli* typically found in hospital settings.

The oils work to weaken the bacterial cell wall, which damages the cell to let antibiotics in to work their magic.

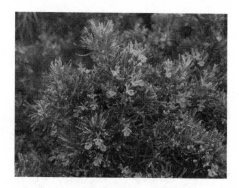

Johns Hopkins' Dr. Nicole M. Parrish says an alternative is sorely needed. She often encounters patients where no antibiotic is effective, a situation which makes her feel helpless as a physician. Parrish says that essential oils are some of the most potent antimicrobial fighters on the planet, and it is crucial to further that understanding to bring about a new class of drugs.

Here are some of the top antibacterial essential oils.

- <u>Cinnamon oil</u> has been shown to be an effective antibacterial agent. In a dental study, it was effective against a type of common bacteria *E. faecalis* that people are susceptible to after having a root canal. The oil eliminated the bacteria altogether by eradicating its biofilm. The oil has also been used agriculturally to fight bacteria in strawberry plants.

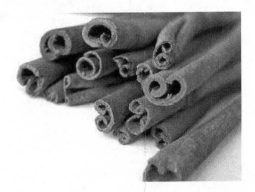

- <u>Thyme</u> is another effective antimicrobial shown to be effective against salmonella commonly found in milk of dairy cattle.

- <u>Oregano</u> has long been used to fight respiratory bacterial infections and is now being used to fight antibiotic resistant infections. Oregano studies have shown the oil to be very effective against certain drug-resistant bacterial strains by disruption of the bacterial cell structure and function.

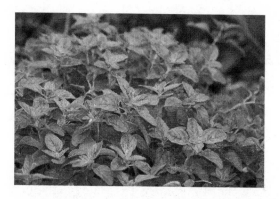

- <u>Tea tree oil</u> has long been used as a topical ointment for skin infections. New research shows that tea tree oil was very effective against staphylococcus and *E. coli*. After the oil was applied, it had an immediate effect on these bacteria, and continued to whittle away for 24 hours.

Antifungal

Fungal infections are very hard to kill. That's because a fungus is similar to human cells. Genes are similar and so are cellular processes, so when you try to kill a fungus, it often ends up impacting the human in a very detrimental way. While there are many antibiotics on the market today to kill bacteria, which are relatively easy to kill, there are only three classes of antifungal drugs. Furthermore, fungi are becoming readily resistant to these drugs.

The only real difference between a human cell and a fungal cell is that the fungus has something called chitin in its cell wall; humans do not. Other organisms also have chitin—organisms like nematodes and protozoa. Most organisms that have chitin end up being pathogens to other species like humans. Chitin is a protein, and under normal circumstances, the human immune system recognizes chitin as a foreign invader and the body deals with it. Cells in the lungs and gastrointestinal tract have chitin receptors to sense an invasion and activate the immune system. Skin does as well. However, sometimes a person's immune response is not functioning properly, so the body cannot clear itself of the chitin. A great example is when a person is allergic to dust mites, which have chitin in their exoskeletons. The person's lungs do not properly detect the mites' chitin, and an allergy develops.

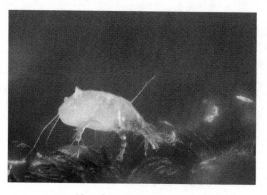

Photo by Gilles San Martin

For this reason, fungal infections are opportunistic, often affecting people with other diseases and compromised immune systems. Chemicals have been shown to be largely ineffective for killing fungi, but essential oils are very promising in fighting these invaders. Here's how they accomplish that.

Fungi form biofilms that help them remain hardy in the host environment. These biofilms help them strongly attach to healthy human cells, and the biofilm also provides an extra support matrix for the cell wall.

Scientists who have studied biofilms show that they provide a protective shield against the human environment, like a layer of extra protection, making them even harder to eradicate. In a medical setting, when a fungus forms its biofilm, it helps the fungus adhere to urinary catheters and other medical apparatus. Once they're on the equipment, they can easily gain access to the bloodstream or urinary organs. Yeast is such a fungus, explaining why so many people in the hospital also develop secondary yeast infections. Once the fungi develop the biofilm, they become even more resistant to antifungal drugs. Research on biofilms is relatively new and there are still many things that scientists don't know about how they work, but they do know that once fungi cells are inside a biofilm, these cells actually communicate with each other for group survival. It's a little creepy, but it shows how hardy the fungi truly are. As the biofilm gains strength, it begins resisting the human body's natural defenses, which over time become less and less effective against the fungus.

Essential oils show promise because they break down the fortress wall of a biofilm. Some drugs do this too, but then they don't kill the fungi inside the biofilm. Essential oils do both. For example, tea tree oil (melaleuca) is very effective against the yeast species Candida albicans; it not only bores through the biofilm, it keeps new fungal cells from forming. Other oils like cinnamon appear to keep the biofilm from forming in the first place. In other trials of the *Mentha suaveolens* plant which is native to Morocco, the essential oil of the plant was found to shut down the metabolic factory of the fungus cells by about 80 percent, rendering them virtually inactive and greatly impaired. Citronella oil is another well-known antifungal oil.

Essential oils are also effective in treating a "super biofilm" called a polymicrobial biofilms, formed by a mixture of bacteria and fungi. These biofilms often occur in patients with chronic infections, and oils like clove, eucalyptus and peppermint have proven effective.

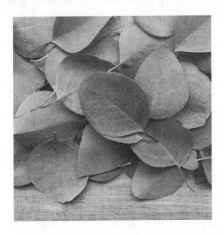

In some trials, eucalyptus has performed better than the common antifungal drug fluconazole. Lemongrass essential oil seems to deform and shrink fungus cells. Anise oil was found to be very effective against a particular type of filamentous fungus, and other oils are found to alter structures and functions inside the fungal cells.

Many plants have two oils that work synergistically together to help or protect the plant, and researchers have found that they continue to work that way in humans. For example, oregano and thyme oil by themselves are great antifungal agents. Researchers have determined that they're even more effective when they work together. They've isolated the compounds carvacrol and thymol in each oil, and when put together cause much more damage to the cell membrane, block toxin production from the fungal cells, and can even cause death of the fungus.

Unfortunately, more and more people are getting fungal infections. The main culprit is *candida* yeast because people are eating more sugar and processed foods that serve as a breeding ground for *candida*. Furthermore, antibiotic overuse creates more fungal infections as they become drug resistant just like bacteria do.

Fungal infections are the cause of so many pesky ailments like toenail fungus, jock itch, vaginal infections and body odor.

However, these essential oils can come to your rescue.

- Lavender has been compared to the antifungal drug clotrimazole for vaginal yeast infections, and researchers found that after 48 hours, there was no difference between the two. This means that given sufficient time, lavender can be effective against these infections.

- Thyme is effective against several different strains of gut bacteria and fungi.

- Peppermint is a well-known oil for stomach upset and it was recently tested against 12 fungal strains and was effective on 11 of them.

- Geranium has been used for centuries to promote healthy skin. It was also an oil that was able to stop or slow the growth of 12 fungal strains tested.

- Bitter almond must be used with extreme caution in humans, but it has been shown to be very effective for agricultural use against 19 common fungal strains that affect crops. It shows promise as a natural pesticide.

- Black pepper is high in antioxidants. Scientists have isolated the chemical compounds in the oil of the pepper plant Piper divaricatum and found strong antifungal agents that are effective even when administered in very low doses.

- Cinnamon has been used since ancient times as an antiviral and antiparasitic agent, but now that scientists have isolated its compounds, it is also shown to be an antifungal and antimicrobial.

- Citronella is well known as a mosquito and insect repellent, but it is also very effective against respiratory infections and was recently found to be effective against seven separate fungal strains.

- Clove helps in gum disease and treats acne, but it is also very effective against candida strains. Clove practically wipes candida out!

- Eucalyptus has helped asthma and pneumonia sufferers for years. The oil is commonly found in products to treat the common cold. The oil is also a very effective antifungal.

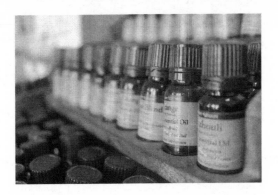

Antiviral

Hundreds of published studies show essential oil effectiveness against viruses. Oils are "fat friendly" and since our cell membranes are lined with fats, the oils easily pass through.

Viruses wreak so much havoc in the human body because they have a tough outer shell called a capsid that protects the virus once it enters the human host. This is why influenza, called an enveloped virus, affects so many people each year. Furthermore, viruses use their own cell walls to fuse with healthy human cell walls in a kind of cellular takeover of the healthy cell. Once they do that, the virus easily replicates.

Oils like lavender and melissa have been shown to inactivate that tough outer coating. The oils either break down the virus cell wall so that it can't fuse to a human cell, or the oils prevent the virus from replicating.

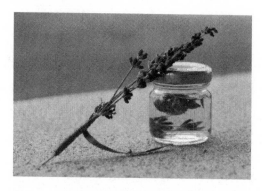

Interestingly, scientists have isolated the active compounds in the oils and have tested that isolated compound as well as the whole oil complex against the virus. For example, tea tree oil was tested against its active compound called terpinen-4-ol. Amazingly, for tea tree as well as several other oils studied in a similar fashion, the whole oil worked ten times better than the isolated compound. Although more research is required, scientists think this is due to the synergistic effects of the oil's compounds—two substances that work together and are better than each part used separately.

Immune oil blends are even more effective because they combine several essential oils to fight the virus on all fronts.

Here are a few of the best antiviral oils:

- Peppermint Oil can do a real number on viruses, particularly the herpes virus that causes cold sores. It can also treat symptoms of the virus that causes the common cold—symptoms like sore throat and congestion.

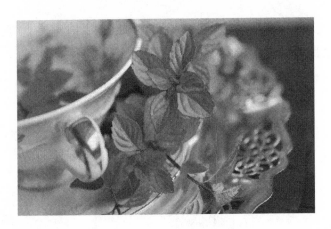

- Thyme Oil kills viruses while at the same time relieving symptoms. It is particularly effective in respiratory infections, as well as herpes virus. It is often used in an immune blend along with cinnamon and clove.

- Rosemary is best known for cooking, but it is very effective against influenza virus, the common cold and herpes viruses.

- Lavender oil is calming but it is also a powerful antiviral agent used to treat the common cold, flu and cold sores.

- Pine oil is a lesser known essential oil that has been tested against multiple strains of the herpes virus with great results. The oil has high levels of antiviral activity, even against drug-resistant viruses.

- Eucalyptus oil is commonly found in over the counter cold remedies, but it is also a powerful antifungal. It works very well on herpes virus cold sores and blisters.

How Do Essential Oils Work?

The chemistry of these essential oils holds the key to how they work. Basically, the oils consist of oxygenated molecules and hydrocarbons that give the oils their effective properties.

Terpenes make up the main hydrocarbon in essential oils. Terpenes are what give the oils their strong aromas. They are present in varying amounts, depending on the oil. For example, the terpene limonene is present in nearly 100 percent concentrations in citrus oils like lemon, wild orange, bergamot and grapefruit. Citronella's terpenes protect it from insects. Every plant has terpenes.

Terpenes are what make a rose smell like a rose and a blueberry smell like a blueberry. Terpenes are secreted by the plant to be attractive to insects for pollination, sticky to trap insects, or pungent to ward off insects. Although terpenes are similar in plant species, they can vary slightly in plants grown in different regions and climates.

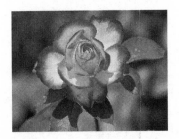

In humans, terpenes are protective to the cells. They help promote cell growth and have great antioxidant qualities. When the oil is absorbed through the skin, it is the terpenes that bind to your cell or brain receptors to create the effects that oil is known for.

Terpenes can be subdivided into smaller groups. Monoterpenes help the cell from building up toxins, and they help support the DNA in every cell. Citrus oils as well as oils like pine, cedar and balsam are high in monoterpenes.

Sesquiterpenes are another subgroup. These are the largest group of terpenes, and they give the oils their thickness. Cells have memory, and sesquiterpenes help to filter out bad information from cellular memory. Oils like myrrh, sandalwood and cedarwood have high levels of sesquiterpenes.

Phenolics are another important compound found in essential oils. They function as "housekeepers" to make sure receptor sites on cells are clean and able to bind to important chemicals. They work with sesquiterpenes by cleaning the receptor first, which allows the sesquiterpenes to then bind to the cell to do their work. Phenolics also have antioxidant properties. Tea tree, wintergreen and clove oils are high in phenolics.

Certain essential oils are high in alcohols, which give the cell its oxidation resistance. They also help the cell to function normally. Geranium and rosewood oils are high in alcohols.

Are Essential Oils Safe?

Most essential oils are safe when used properly. Anytime you're introduced to something new, it's a good idea to proceed conservatively, and the same is true with oils.

Essential oils are classified as GRAS or Generally Recognized As Safe by the U.S. Food and Drugs Administration (FDA). Very few people have adverse side effects when these oils are properly used. There are several factors to keep in mind.

Dosage

Just as with medication, dosage is a very important part of essential oil safety. Using oil in high doses can do harm; for example, they can cause a skin reaction if used topically and incorrectly.

Dose is important to follow regardless of how you're using the oil, whether aromatically, topically, or internally.

Remember that an essential oil dose will always depend on the age, size, health status, and personal skin sensitivity of the individual. If you have specific concerns about your skin, it is always a good idea to consult with your physician before using essential oils topically.

Dose will vary depending on your health status, age and weight. When using an essential oil for the first time, always start with the lowest possible dose, around one or two drops, see how your body reacts to the small dose, then increase over time according to package directions.

It is important to always remember that oils are very concentrated and thus very potent. So, it is better to use a few small doses periodically throughout the day instead of using or taking a single large dose.

Most aromatherapy oil-based blends of more than one oil are between one and five percent dilutions, so they don't pose a safety risk.

Application Methods

Some oils can be used aromatically, topically and ingested, while others have a specific single application. Always follow directions. Some oils are safe topically, but cause issues when inhaled, and vice versa.

Before you use an oil, make sure you know its recommended application method, as well as the concentration and dosage. Never ingest oils without professional guidance.

Since most essential oils cannot be applied directly to the skin without dilution, don't forget to use your carrier oil.

Sensitivity

All people are different—with different chemical compositions, health status and makeups. Therefore, it is possible for any oil to cause sensitivity. Children are more likely to have a sensitivity response so extra safety precautions should be taken. Oils are generally not a good idea for children under age seven.

You can apply an oil topically as a form of sensitivity test when first using the oil. Use one drop with a carrier oil and see how your skin reacts. Check the test area every hour.

Some oils can slightly change composition if exposed to the sun or UV light, because their compounds are photosensitive. Citrus oils, in particular, have this issue, but oil manufacturers will usually post it on the label. The light sensitivity can change the oil and you might become more sun-sensitive as a result. The potency of oil can affect children. Some oils should be avoided altogether, while others should only be used in a highly diluted form and under the guidance of a knowledgeable professional. For example, wintergreen and birch should never be used on children due to the high concentrations of methyl salicylate.

Purity

Always make sure to use pure essential oils. There are some imposters on the market that contain alterations like addition of synthetic chemicals or dilutions with vegetable oil. The label should indicate purity. Note that some expensive oils like rose oil (at $100 a teaspoon) are sometimes sold in diluted form, but it will be advertised on the label.

Just know that oils that are not pure have an increased likelihood of creating an adverse response, so it is very important to only buy pure and genuine essential oils.

Drug Interactions

Not much research has been done on interactions of essential oils with standard pharmaceutical drugs, but it does make sense that it could happen, due to the complex chemical nature of the oils.

It's always important, if you're on prescription medications, to talk over use of any new product with your doctor. More research is being done every day, like a study showing that peppermint and eucalyptus oils increase the skin absorption of the anti-cancer drug called 5-fluorouracil.

Certain oils are known to interact with blood thinner medications, like clary sage, cypress, eucalyptus, ginger, rosemary, sage and thyme.

Toxicity

Rarely does a toxic event occur with appropriate use of essential oils. Toxicity is typically due to misuse or accidental ingestion of an oil, particularly by children.

There are some oils that have been banned by The International Fragrance Association which monitors the industry. They've banned certain essential oils because they have been found to be toxic when ingested or applied topically: cade oil crude, costus root, elecampane, fig leaf absolute, horseradish, nightshade, pennyroyal, rue, sassafras, savin, southernwood, stinging nettle, stryax gum, tea absolute, wormseed and wormwood.

How Are Essential Oils Produced?

Oils must be extracted from the plant parts and bottled effectively as a product. There are several methods for producing and extracting essential oils.

Distillation

Steam distillation is a common method for extracting essential oils from plants. The plant parts are put onto a grid and boiling water is placed underneath. As the steam rises, the oils are literally pulled out of the plant. The steam and the oil rise together and it is captured in a jar-like container and drained using tubing. The oil/water mixture is rapidly cooled and since water and oils don't mix, the two are separated and the oil is collected. Depending on the oil, the remaining water can sometimes contain some of the aromatic compounds of the plant. This water by-product is called a hydrosol and is very fragrant and used in cosmetic products.

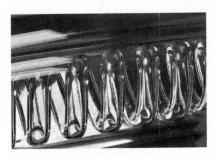

Expression

Expression is the most direct way to extract an essential oil. This method involves pressing the oil-containing plant parts—leaves, seeds, flowers, skins—in a process very similar to how olive oil is made. For example, expression is used on citrus rinds to press the oil out of the skins.

Carbon Dioxide

Extraction of oils using carbon dioxide (CO_2) is a relatively new and interesting process that has been around for approximately 10 years. It is a very expensive process, but results in a very high quality oil. Compressed CO_2 is used in a high pressure, low temperature process to extract the oil from botanicals.

Solvents

While chemical solvents can be used to extract oils from the plants, most producers prefer not to use this method out of concern that trace elements of the chemicals will be left behind. In this method, the plant is completely dissolved in solvents like benzene or methylene. Then the solvent is removed via evaporation using a vacuum or centrifuge device to pull the solvent from the essential oil. The oil product that results is called an "absolute". This process is very expensive, and usually reserved for expensive oils which can't be distilled (rose, vanilla, jasmine).

Enfleurage

Enfleurage is a very old traditional method only used in France today because it requires a high skill level and is complicated and very expensive. Flower blossoms are placed in warm fat that absorbs the oil out of the flowers. The French used to use lard or animal fat but now use vegetable fats in the process. The flowers are then removed and the process is repeated several times. Once enough oil is in the fats, the two are separated to leave just the essential oil product.

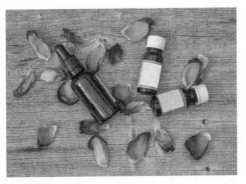

How To Use Essential Oils

Essential oils can be used in many versatile ways: aromatic, topical and even by internal ingestion. Each oil has an ideal use or can perhaps be used in all these ways. As scientists conduct more research, they're developing a greater understanding of application methods specific to each oil.

Oils have amazing physical and emotional wellness applications. You can use single oils, or a complex blend of oils specially formulated for specific health applications, such as mood enhancing or respiratory. Let's explore some of the ways oils can be used.

Aromatic

Because they are volatile, and thus change state from solid to gas quickly, essential oils rapidly disperse through the air, so they're excellent for aromatherapy applications.

One of the most popular uses for essential oils is aromatherapy for emotional wellness. The receptors in our noses (olfactory receptors) quickly absorb the oil's scent. The olfactory nerve sends that signal to the limbic system, a part of the brain responsible for emotions, memory and behavior. In this process, hormones are released in your body. Think back to the last time you smelled roses; perhaps it evoked a memory of the person who brought you the bouquet, or a memory of playing in your grandmother's rose garden as a child. These are examples of your limbic system at work.

Some essential oils like citrus oils (grapefruit, orange, lemon or bergamot) are uplifting and invigorating, as are oils like peppermint and rosemary. Other oils like lavender and chamomile are calming. You may have had chamomile tea to calm yourself before bedtime; using chamomile oil is the same concept. The oils stimulate physical and emotional responses because the oils affect your mood and emotions. You'll likely be drawn to your favorite aromas instinctively.

The easiest way to do aromatherapy is to put a few drops of oil in your hands, rub them together, cup your hands over your nose and inhale the delicious aroma.

Diffusers

As this is not always practical, many people use a device called a diffuser. Using a diffuser is one of the easiest ways to use oils aromatically.

Terra cotta: There are some inexpensive diffuser options, like terra cotta jars or discs, a dish and candle or an electric plug-in scent pad. Terra-cotta is the burnt orange pottery you think of when you think of a regular flower pot.

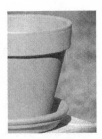

The ceramic material is porous, so using a terra cotta container filled with oil means the oil will seep through the walls and infuse the air with scent. You can also buy sticks with terra cotta tops. Get a small glass jar and fill with oil. The oil will seep up the wooden sticks into the terra cotta tops and fill the air with aroma.

Some people even wear terra cotta pendants like a necklace; the back is glazed to prevent oil from getting on your skin or clothing. Larger terra cotta disks are available and work the same as the pendant. Think of it as a coaster you can infuse with oil! The back is glazed to prevent oil from leaking onto your furniture.

A terra cotta diffuser is a great way to get the oil aroma without using any powered device—just know that the oils disperse continuously. In short, there's no off switch. You can always put the disc in a plastic bag if you don't want the aroma at certain times.

A terra cotta diffuser is best used with the same oil. Switch to another oil only after the first oil is completely evaporated. Otherwise the oils will mix and may produce an unpleasant smell.

Candle diffuser: A candle diffuser is also a simple method of aromatherapy. A dish containing water and a few drops of oil sits on top of a candle, which provides the heat to diffuse the oil. Since essential oils don't dissolve in water, this is an effective way to scent a room. The candle is enough to heat but not boil the water, so the oils evaporate. Always use water and not oil directly, and keep an eye on the water as it evaporates so that you are not heating an empty dish. These oils are called volatile for a reason; they will quickly burn onto the surface of the dish, likely ruining your diffuser and creating a burnt aroma—not what you were going for at all! Just know that essential oils should never be directly burned. This is very dangerous, and direct burning changes the chemical structure of the oil so that it is no longer affected.

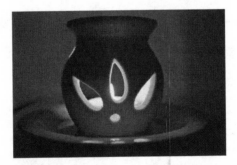

You can reuse a candle diffuser; just make sure you've thoroughly washed the dish before you use a different oil. If oils have ever burned onto the dish and can't be easily cleaned, you might not be able to reuse the dish. Certainly, over time, the dish will wear out and you'll have to buy a new dish to go with the candle diffuser. Within time, the dish, but not the whole diffuser, will need to be replaced.

As with all candles, safety is important. Never leave a candle diffuser unattended and never use overnight due to fire risk. Many people use essential oils at night as a sleep remedy, but a candle diffuser is not a good option for this use.

Electric Diffusers: An electric diffuser is a good option for anytime and anywhere you want to use oils. They don't involve an open flame and are much safer. However, they do require power: battery, plug in or USB. Some diffusers come with all three options. This is the best option for overnight use because it does not require constant monitoring.

The best way to use oils for inhalation is to purchase an essential oils diffuser. Water is placed in the device along with a few drops of a single oil or more than one oil to create an oil blend. The diffuser creates a fine mist vapor. It's a great way to scent a room.

Electric diffusers use cool water in a chamber. You add a few drops of oil to the water and the device makes a cool mist that fills the room. There are many inexpensive options on the market. Some are battery-powered, so they're transportable to use anywhere, and some have USB cables to run off your computer or even in your car. And speaking of your car, there are even smaller options that plug into a USB or lighter outlet. Many diffusers have an automatic shutoff option, so when the device runs out of water, the motor shuts off so as to not burn out the unit.

This type of diffuser can give you a wider disbursement of aroma because the vapor mist more easily fills the room. Most diffusers require about a cup of water with about 5 drops of oil directly added to the water. You can add different oils, such as orange, lemon and grapefruit for a citrus powerhouse!

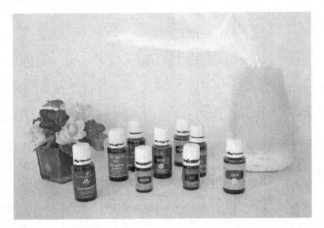

Electric diffusers are generally safe. They release small amounts of vapor into the air and are very unlikely to cause the concentration of any essential oil to rise to unsafe levels. If the fragrance is too intense, raise a window to ventilate the room.

Diffusers should generally be used for about 30 minutes at a time, and try to avoid leaving your diffuser plugged in overnight. You can purchase a diffuser that has an automatic shutoff in case you forget to turn it off.

Because they are flammable, keep all oils and diffusers away from open flames. Don't overfill your diffuser, and never add carrier oils as it will gunk up the mechanism. Because diffusers use water, you're not required to add a carrier oil.

To keep your diffuser working properly, periodically wash it with soap and warm water. If stagnant water is left sitting, mold can grow, particularly in humid environments, and you certainly don't want to be misting mold into your home.

On a related note, essential oils should never be added to a humidifier, which are not made for this purpose.

Other Aromatherapy Methods

Aromatherapy is certainly not a new concept. It's been practiced for thousands of years. If you don't have a diffuser readily available, there are lots of other ways you can enjoy aromatherapy.

Dry evaporation: place oil on a cotton ball and allow it to evaporate into the air. Some people even put oil-infused cotton balls inside their car air vents for a fresh interior.

Steam: Add drops of essential oil to a steaming bowl of water. This can serve as a mini-facial spa treatment if you let the steam open your pores. Or you can place a towel over the bowl, put your head under it, and inhale the vapors. Please realize this is a very intense, direct way to inhale oils so one or two drops is enough. Lots of people use a steam containing eucalyptus essential oil to relieve nasal congestion.

Personal inhaler: You can purchase either a plastic inhaler or aluminum inhaler. Both have a wick and you can add essential oil to it, then cap for later use. Anytime you need a boost, uncap and waft under your nose. Most inhalers last a few months; just refill with oil when you feel it's lost its effectiveness.

Smelling salts: Along the same lines as the personal inhaler, you can make your own smelling salts. Just use 1 tablespoon of rock salt with 10 drops of your favorite oil. Store the mixture in a tightly-sealed container and use whenever you need a boost of clear thought.

Spray: Purchase a small sprayer bottle, add water and drops of essential oil, shake, and you have just made your own air freshener. Make sure the bottle is set for a fine mist spray. Lots of people spray the air or spray fabric furniture or rugs to freshen them up. You can also do it for curtains and comforters, or even use as a disinfecting spray by choosing an antibacterial oil to spray on kitchen counters, yoga mats, pet areas and other places where germs like to hide.

Add oil to other products: Add oil to your laundry detergent or dryer sheets for an added boost. You can even add oils to a cool light bulb (emphasis on cool). As the bulb heats, the aroma disperses. Or, ceramic round donut-shaped diffuser rings are specifically made for this purpose. You put the oil on the ring and slip the ceramic over the light bulb.

Perfume: many believers in essential oil even make their own perfume. Mix 25 drops of oil with an ounce of either perfume alcohol or denatured alcohol. Depending on the oil you choose, you might also need a carrier oil which is discussed below. Sweet almond oil or coconut oil are good choices for perfume carrier oils.

Best Aromatherapy Oils

Relaxation: for relaxation, lavender is frequently used, as is chamomile. Use this in the evening to calm your busy mind before sleep.

Sleep: Marjoram oil is another wonderful sleep-inducing oil.

Congestion: eucalyptus, peppermint or juniper are great for stuffy noses. There are even respiratory blend oils you can buy that are already mixed for you.

Skin: Tea tree oil in a steam facial can work wonders for skin problems.

Energy: Lots of people swear by citrus oils to get them up and going for the day. These oils are great mood boosters.

Cleaner: for a fresh clean scent all around your house, use lemon.

Holidays: spray pine, peppermint or clove oil for the holiday spirit.

Is Aromatherapy Safe?

Now that you know about different diffuser types, aromatherapy methods and oils, you might be wondering if it is safe to inhale essential oils. Indirect methods are very safe, but direct inhalation right out of the bottle, or by the steam or personal inhaler method warrant a few cautions.

First, these direct methods are not recommended for pregnant women or children under age 7. If you're steaming under a towel, either close your eyes or wear protective gear like swim goggles to protect your eyes. Some oils are very potent.

It is also recommended that you not use eucalyptus oil if you have asthma. Instead, pine oil is a safer substitute. Always consult your doctor.

Inhalation of oils remains a very low risk level to most people. The concentration of oil in the room is unlikely to ever get to a dangerous level. If you have prolonged exposure to highly oil-concentrated vapor—exposure of more than an hour—you might feel sluggish or have headaches, dizziness or nausea.

Topical

Topical application of essential oils is fast, simple, and effective. Used topically, oils are soothing in massage and excellent for the skin. With topical application, you can target specific areas of your body.

Molecules in the oil penetrate the skin and seep into tissues, muscles and joints. They easily penetrate the skin because they're lipid soluble, and once through, they stay in the local area to provide their benefits. As you might imagine, topical application is very effective.

Oils can calm, moisturize, reduce inflammation and help your cells eliminate waste products.

Oils are easily absorbed, but you can increase absorption by lightly massaging the area to stimulate blood flow.

Carrier Oils

You can also use an oil called a carrier oil to not only increase absorption but to help dilute stronger oils that may cause skin irritation when applied topically. Carrier oils can also help to slow the evaporation rate of the oil on your skin.

Oils like basil, oregano and tea tree are very strong, and applied alone, can cause skin sensitivity. One of the most common and popular carrier oils is fractionated coconut oil. The term "fractionated" refers to a fraction of the coconut oil components being used in this application. This oil is a fraction of the whole, virgin coconut oil that is harvested.

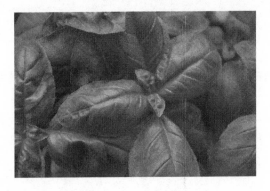

Fractionation tends to prolong the oil's shelf life. Many vegetable oils can oxidize and spoil over time. Discard your oil if it smells rancid.

The dilution is typically a 1:3 ratio—one drop of essential oil to three drops of coconut oil. Dilution is very important when using essential oils. Don't worry—use of fractionated coconut oil or another carrier oil will not minimize the essential oil benefits. In fact, it makes the situation better by increasing the absorption and extending the benefits.

Although coconut oil is the most common carrier oil, it's not the only one. Any pure vegetable oil is a good carrier oil because these oils can easily dissolve an essential oil without disrupting the oil's effectiveness.

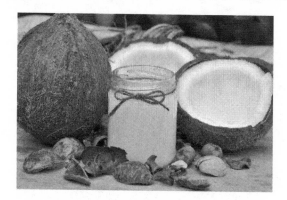

The following oils are also very commonly used as carrier oils because they are lightweight and non-greasy:

- Avocado oil
- Walnut oil
- Macadamia nut oil
- Sweet almond oil
- Linseed oil
- Sunflower oil
- Olive oil
- Apricot kernel oil
- Jojoba oil
- Grapeseed oil

Here are some examples of oils that always need to be diluted:

- Cassia
- Cinnamon
- Clove
- Cumin
- Geranium
- Lemongrass
- Oregano
- Thyme

You will typically find common carrier oils available for purchase in natural foods stores. It's preferable to buy carrier oils that are organic and cold-pressed. Most carrier oils do not have a strong smell, so they don't mask the scent of the essential oil you are using. Ideally, keep your carrier oils refrigerated; they'll typically keep a year.

Topical use is a great essential oil application; since the VACs are so small, they easily pass through the skin into the bloodstream.

Skin

Many oils cleanse and purify and as such, have long been used to keep skin healthy. Oils are commonly used to soothe irritated skin and to help heal skin imperfections like acne.

Many modern skincare products contain chemicals, but essential oils are natural, free from fillers, chemicals and even toxins present in today's cleaners, toners and other skin products.

Oils can be used by people who have very sensitive skin who typically struggle to find a skincare product that won't cause a reaction. Instead, oils can simply be diluted to accommodate sensitive skin.

Lots of people make their own beauty and skin care remedies from essential oils. Here are a few ideas:

- Add geranium to your existing facial moisturizer. It will provide your skin with a healthy glow.
- Make your own body butter lotion with coconut oil, shea butter and essential oils.

- Use coconut oil, beeswax and lavender oil for a yummy and healing lip balm.
- Soothe your feet after a long day with a large basin of warm water and some lemon and eucalyptus oils.
- Some ladies swear by this cellulite remedy of coconut oil mixed with a few drops of grapefruit seed essential oil
- Create your own perfume with jasmine or ylang-ylang oil. Lavender and vanilla are great for women, and cypress and clove are great for men's natural chemistry.
- Make your own face wash with raw honey and tea tree oil. It's great for acne.
- Create a facial sugar scrub with sugar (or rock salt) and almond oil plus an essential oil of your choice.
- Make a natural skin toner with a cup of water, and two drops each of lavender, geranium and frankincense oils.
- To strengthen fingernails, use vitamin E and add lemon, frankincense and myrrh; rub on nails and cuticles

- Use sandalwood, geranium, lavender and frankincense essential oils with an unscented lotion as a great wrinkle reducer (avoid the eye area)
- Frankincense essential oil applied directly to sun spots and age spots can dramatically reduce their appearance
- Use coconut oil mixed with frankincense and myrrh and grapefruit seed essential oils to reduce stretch marks.
- Heal your dry, cracked feet by mixing coconut oil and lavender; apply to feet, wear socks overnight, and you'll wake up with soft and supple tootsies!

If you're going to have five oils on hand for skin and beauty, pick these:
- Calm irritated skin – lavender and Roman chamomile
- Reduce age spots – frankincense
- Thicken hair – rosemary and sage
- Natural SPF skin protection – helichrysum and myrrh
- Acne and blemishes - melaleuca (tea tree) and geranium

Body

Adding a few drops of oil to a warm bath can soak tired muscles and calm your senses. Lavender is a popular bath additive. Since oils are not water soluble, they'll float on top of the water, which is great for aromatherapy but not so great for skin absorption. Use a few tablespoons of whole milk or cream to act as a dispersant for the oil. This will ensure it is evenly spread throughout your bath water. Bath salts can also be used to disperse essential oils. Try this recipe: three parts sea salt, two parts Epsom salt and one part baking soda; add to that a few drops of your favorite oil.

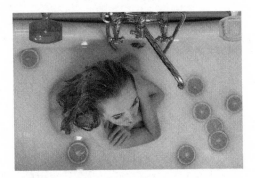

Massage is one of the oldest topical uses of essential oil. You can massage body, feet, hands or any area that is sore and will benefit from massage. Therapists usually use about six drops of essential oil mixed with a carrier oil. Massaging the neck, forehead, temples, arms, legs, feet and hands with essential oils can be extremely relaxing.

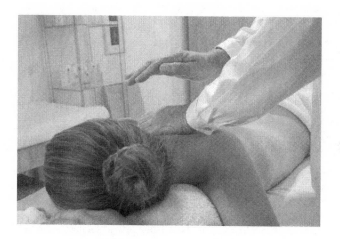

If you sit for long hours at your desk, and you have tension in your neck and shoulders, consider an essential oils massage to unwind.

Some people apply oils topically to the chest to promote breathing and clear congestion.

Hot or cold compresses can be made by adding essential oils for their soothing properties.

If you've got sore muscles from a workout or joint pain from arthritis, you can use essential oils to soothe pain.

Many oil manufacturers make oil pain blends. Many essential oils have cooling and warming properties, which help sore muscles.

You might have been instructed to apply oils on the bottoms of your feet. When first trying an oil, the bottom of the feet are a great starting point. The pores are larger, the skin is much thicker and less sensitive. Try it out! Lots of people place the oils on their feet prior to bedtime.

Have you ever had an upset stomach? Use a few drops of peppermint oil with coconut oil for a belly rub; it helps to calm your digestion and your upset stomach.

Hair

Adding essential oils to your hair products is a great way to provide extra moisture or deal with problems like an itchy, dry scalp. For example, rosemary can invigorate the scalp tissue. There are many hair care products on the market that already contain essential oils, such as argan oil for extra moisturizing.

Essential oils like lavender, sage and rosemary stimulate the scalp and hair follicles and can naturally thicken hair and help with hair loss. Hormone levels affect hair loss, and lavender and clary sage help to balance estrogen levels. Likewise, rosemary stops the hormone known as dihydroxy-testosteron or DHT, and therefore stops hair loss.

Here are some tried-and-true home remedies:
- A scalp massage oil made of 10 drops of rosemary oil and 5 drops of lavender oil
- A natural shampoo of coconut milk, aloe vera gel and lavender and rosemary oils
- Addition of lavender, cedarwood or basil essential oils to your shampoo to reduce itching
- A mix of unscented oil plus rosemary and lavender essential oils as a scalp massage for dandruff
- Rosemary oil added to shampoo to thicken hair and add volume
- Unscented oil mixed with sandalwood and lavender essential oils as a hair conditioner
- Ylang ylang, rosemary and lime oils mixed with unscented oil as a scalp massage for oily hair.

Gargle

Add essential oils to water to use as a gargle. Wintergreen and peppermint freshen breath and clove can help heal gums. In fact, when people develop a complication known as dry socket from wisdom tooth extraction surgery, a clove packet is put into the empty tooth socket. Patients feel immediate relief. Gargling with clove oil can have the same effect for inflamed gums. In fact, there are essential oil mouthwashes on the market; they contain a heavy amount of clove oil for gum healing. If you have a sore throat, gargle with tea tree oil. Whatever oil you use, it only takes a few drops in warm water. Do not swallow the gargle mixture.

Bug Spray

You can even make your own homemade, all natural bug spray and avoid chemicals like toxic DEET in commercial mosquito repellent products. All of the oils below repel insects. You can spray or rub them on to put insects at bay.

- Citronella
- Lemongrass
- Eucalyptus

- Peppermint
- Clove

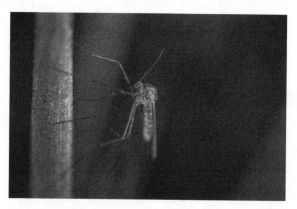

Best Topical Oils

Here are just a few of the literally hundreds of topical uses for essential oils.

- Basil: Apply to the temples and neck to reduce tension
- Bergamot: Apply to the skin during your shower for skin-purifying benefits
- Black Pepper: Apply to your feet for a stimulating wake up
- Clary Sage: Apply to your abdomen during your menstrual cycle to help with cramps

- Roman Chamomile: Add to your favorite shampoo or conditioner
- Rose: Rub on face for even skin tone and healthy complexion
- Rosemary: Massage into the scalp
- Vetiver: Use for a foot massage after a long day of standing
- Mint oils (peppermint or wintergreen): place a few drops in hand, rub together, inhale for an energy boost
- Ylang Ylang: place on back of neck to calm and uplift

Topical Safety

For any topical product, you should always use safety precautions. Be sure to look for any irritation that occurs. Follow proper dosage, and use a carrier oil if recommended. Individuals react to essential oils differently, so it's wise to determine how your body will react to the new oil. Once you determine that, proceed with using these beneficial oils.

When essential oils are used topically, there is always the chance for sensitivity or skin irritation. Certain parts of your body, such as nasal tissues, mouth tissue, inner ears and eyes are very sensitive to oils. Be sure to wash your hands of excess oil, and avoid touching your face or rubbing your eyes if you have oil on your fingers.

Elderly people can have more skin sensitivity, particularly to high-menthol oils like eucalyptus and peppermint. The elderly may want to avoid certain oils or only use in a highly diluted form.

Here are oils known to cause skin irritation:

- Bay
- Cinnamon bark or leaf
- Clove bud
- Citronella
- Cumin
- Lemongrass
- Lemon verbena
- Oregano
- Thyme

The use of topical oils during pregnancy remains controversial. The main concern is for oils that can cross from the mother's body through the placenta to affect the baby. It's important to note that just because an oil crosses the placenta does not mean it will cause harm to either the mother or the fetus. Still, there are concerns, particularly about use of oils during the first trimester of pregnancy.

As an example, let's say a mother takes a nightly bath with a few drops of lavender for calming. While it is unlikely that this would cause any problems for the unborn child, use remains controversial.

It is an old wives' tale that use of oils like clary sage or rosemary in either an aromatherapy way or as a massage oil can cause a miscarriage. There are no recorded cases. Pregnant women have to take very large doses of essential oils like pennyroyal which then become a toxic dose.

Indeed, the occasional use of a few drops of safe oil as part of a bath or massage probably does more good than harm because it relaxes the mother and soothes the discomforts of pregnancy.

Still, there is lack of scientific information regarding oil use during pregnancy, so it is best to adhere to general safety guidelines regarding the oils and to check with your doctor prior to starting any use.

People with damaged, diseased, or inflamed skin are much more likely to be sensitive to oils and have skin reactions. Never use an undiluted oil on damaged or diseased skin because you may worsen the skin condition. Also, when skin is diseased, a larger than normal amount of oil might be absorbed.

Just remember that when it comes to topical use, it's better to use several small doses throughout the day rather than a single large dose. Small doses can be repeated every few hours.

Internal Ingestion

Certain essential oils can be ingested internally as dietary supplements. This is not a new concept; you essentially already do this—every time you have mint in your tea, cinnamon on your toast or basil on your pasta.

Because oils are in a concentrated form, they can be ingested to have targeted and potent effects on your health.

Internal use is safe and effective; once ingested, essential oils directly enter the blood stream through the gastrointestinal tract. Once there, they are transported throughout the rest of the body, and because they are soluble in lipids, all organs easily uptake and use them, including the brain.

Just like other nutrients we intake, oils are metabolized by the liver and then excreted as a waste product.

Proper dosing is particularly important when ingesting oils. Lots of oils users take essential oils internally in a veggie capsule or mix it with a bit of water or yogurt.

See the culinary uses of oil section for oils to use when cooking.

Ingestion Safety

The best rule of thumb is to never ingest an essential oil without professional advice from a practitioner or aromatherapist. A licensed individual will have certification from The Alliance of International Aromatherapists (AIA) or alternative agency. Just because someone sells essential oils does not mean they are a licensed professional, so beware.

The AIA does not endorse any internal use of oils unless recommended by a clinically trained health practitioner (doctor, nurse, etc.) for safety reasons.

Furthermore, there is not enough research on how essential oils interact with the gut's natural flora, meaning the roughly four pounds of healthy bacteria that lives in your digestive tract. It is unsure how each oil affects that bacteria and whether it contributes or detracts from the healthy flora balance.

There's no scientific support to say that essential oils only kill harmful bacteria; they may kill the beneficial gut bacteria too. Significantly more research is needed in this area.

Certainly, many oils have antibacterial qualities, but effects on gut bacteria are unknown at this time. There is some evidence to indicate that oils might be effective. Peppermint oil coated do help with inflammatory bowel disease; in one study, the oil did help the balance of beneficial gut bacteria.

Last but not least, for most oils, ingestion is not the most effective method. Ingestion is the right application only in very specific situations, so try to stick to aromatic and topical uses.

Oils have an effect on internal tissues and the delicate mucosal lining in the esophagus and other tissues, particularly in the digestive tract. Some studies show that certain oils, like citrus oils, contain limonene which might have a protective effect on mucosal tissues, but again, it is too early and there is not enough conclusive research, so erring on the side of caution is best.

Oils that should never be ingested internally are:

- Basil
- Birch
- Black pepper
- Cardamom
- Cedarwood
- Citronella
- Eucalyptus
- Melaleuca (Tea Tree)

How do I choose the best method to apply essential oils?

The application method chosen depends on the desired effect and the essential oil selected, but moreso, it depends on the labeled use of the oil, so follow those labels! For example, some essential oils are irritating to the skin because of their chemistry. These would need more dilution or might better be used by inhalation.

Here are some use tips:

- Topical applications are best for skin conditions and wound care.

- Use aromatherapy to lighten your mood.

- Taking a bath gives you a double dip, so to speak, since it involves topical absorption and aromatherapy.

If you're not sure how to use your new essential oils, consult a qualified aromatherapist.

What conditions can be treated with essential oils?

Anxiety, depression, and stress

Aromatherapy is a real, effective therapy for mood disorders like depression and anxiety. Have you ever had chamomile tea at night to calm down? The essential oils of the plant are in the tea. They work, don't they? In a recent study conducted in China, scientists performed animal studies involving aromatherapy using Roman chamomile essential oil for two weeks. Amazingly, scientists used imaging to show the inhalation of the VACs "light up" in the hippocampus, the part of the animal's brain that regulates mood.

Certain essential oils like those in the mint family (spearmint, peppermint and others) contain the chemical compound carvone. Brazilian scientists published a recent study showing the significant calming effect of carvone on subjects with anxiety.

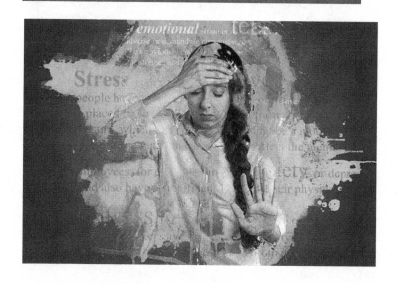

Anxiety is how your body prepares itself to deal with a threatening situation, and in today's stressful world, many experience some degree of anxiety, perhaps even on a daily basis. Over time, this form of stress takes its toll—emotionally and physically. Fear, nervousness and even palpitations are common symptoms. Heart rate and blood pressure both increase.

To soothe anxiety, here are the top essential oils to use:

- Lavender oil is considered a universal oil known for its relaxing effect. Mist your pillow before bedtime or add some to your bath.

- The fresh sharp scent of wild orange oil is very uplifting for both the body and the mind. It is also calming and has been shown to reducing heart palpitations brought on by anxiety.

- Lemon oil can lower blood pressure and calm nerves with its invigorating fragrance.
- Clary sage is actually part of the mint family, and mixed with bergamot oil, calms the nerves.
- Lemon balm helps people with the anxiety caused by an over-active thyroid.

Relaxation

Many of these same oils can be used for simple aromatherapy relaxation. Put a few drops of oil on your hands and rub them together to emit the wonderful smells. Or place oil on a cotton ball and breathe in the aroma. Massage therapists use essential oils during massage; not only are the oils absorbed through the skin, but their aroma is also released into the air for inhalation.

Insomnia

Who among us couldn't use a better night's sleep? Poor sleep has downstream repercussions on many other areas of health. For example, dementia patients are very prone to sleep disturbances. A Japanese study used aromatherapy for a 20-day period; oils were put onto a towel left near the patient's pillow. Subjects slept longer and got better quality of sleep.

Single oils like lavender and chamomile are very effective for sleep, and there are also blended oils designed for sleep that contain lavender, chamomile, and other oils such as cedarwood or vetiver. Here are the best sleep-inducing oils:

- Lavender is most known for being related to sleep. It can be used in a diffuser or as a mist on your pillow. It is so effective that hospital ICUs are starting to use it to help patients sleep.

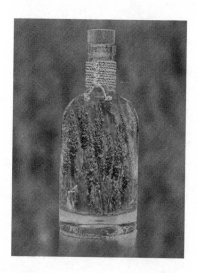

- Vetiver essential oil is distilled from the roots of the plant, so it has a rich, earthy smell. If you want your brain to shut off for a good night's sleep, this is your oil.

- Roman chamomile is best known for its tea possessing calming, soothing, and relaxing properties. Chamomile oil's light, floral scent will get you at peace in no time.

- Ylang Ylang has a fruity and floral scent that can help the quality of your sleep.

- Bergamot is a citrus fruit often added to teas. Bergamot is described as emotional balancing and will definitely help you sleep.

Allergy

Essential oils might be useful in seasonal allergy symptoms. Oils used for respiratory support contain the chemical compound eucalyptol, shown to be very effective in combating the immune system changes that occur with seasonal allergies. Oregano has long been used for respiratory problems, and other oils like cardamom and rosemary are very effective. In a recent study in mice, essential oil compound mixtures showed a great reduction in airway inflammation.

An allergy is an abnormal response by your immune system when it comes into contact with a specific substance known as an allergen. Your body releases histamine for allergens like food, grasses and pollens, mold and pet hair. Essential oils are a great all-natural alternative to medications. Here are the top five:

- Melaleuca (Tea Tree) – to treat mold and fungi allergies.
- Roman Chamomile – great for respiratory problems stemming from allergies.
- Melissa (Lemon Balm) – Melissa is from the mint family and this oil can be inhaled to easy any allergic reaction
- Peppermint – this oil can be applied directly to the skin or diluted to help with pollen and other seasonal allergies. The L-menthol in the oil stops inflammation.

- Lavender – lavender can halt immediate allergic reactions that result in swelling or itching.

Immune System

Our immune systems suffer a daily onslaught of bacteria, viruses and environmental threats. Add in lifestyle factors of stress and poor sleep, and our immune systems usually do not fare well. Immunity has two parts. The first line of defense protects the body from invader entry; the skin and gastrointestinal tract are good examples. If an invader does happen to get past the first line of defense, we have mobilized immunity that comes to the rescue. White blood cells rush to the infection. Boosting both aspects of the immune system is important in order to stay healthy.

Oregano is powerful for respiratory issues. Clove oil has both anti-bacterial and anti-parasite qualities. A protein called chitin is produced by insects as a waste product. People inhale it from the circulating air. Chitin is an example of one of the intruders we are exposed to on a daily basis. Scientists studied the effects of peppermint and thyme essential oils on chitin. Amazingly, these oils reversed the negative respiratory effects of chitin. The chitin is still present in the air—nothing can be done about that—but the oils made the cells not have an adverse reaction to it.

You're probably tempted to run and get antibiotics every time you get a cold, but that won't work because viruses—not bacteria—cause colds. There's no cure for a cold—you just have to tough it out. Rest and stay hydrated. But there are some oils you can add to diffuse through the air, and that might help:

- Eucalyptus has both antibacterial and antiviral properties and is part of many over-the-counter products because of it. It helps to dilate the bronchioles for easy breathing and it can break up the mucus of congestion. Use it if you have congestion or a stuffy nose or cough.

- Cardamom helps ease any stomach upset you might have with the cold.

- Geranium flowers may smell great but the oil also has tremendous antiseptic and antibacterial properties. It's great for disinfecting the air and surfaces in your home, which is very helpful when you have a sick household.

- Lemon is great to have around the house for so many reasons, but it can be particularly effective during illness. Your lymphatic system becomes sluggish when you're ill and this oil can mildly stimulate the lymphatics.

- Peppermint, like cardamom, can soothe stomachs and reduce nausea. It is also great for coughs. It's a real immune-booster.

- Rosemary is mostly known for cooking but it is very helpful for a cough and joint pains that often happen when you have a cold. It also zaps headaches.

Arthritis and Joint Pain

Essential oils can be topically applied right to the muscle or joint to relieve pain. Some of these oils require a carrier oil to help the oil go deep into the tissue. The oils are rapidly absorbed through the skin, so they're a very effective method and natural, anti-inflammatory agent at site of the inflammation that is caused by arthritis.

Several research studies have shown that topical essential oils can be effective against arthritis. Here are the most effective oils.

- Ginger has amazing healing agents that are both analgesic and anti-inflammatory. It decreases pain associated with arthritis by acting on the vanilloid receptors of the sensory nerves. When applied, the ginger oil can have a slight burning sensation, so a carrier oil is recommended. The Arthritis Foundation reported on a study that showed ginger can even substitute for nonsteroidal anti-inflammatory drugs (NSAIDs) like Tylenol. Research has shown that ginger affects inflammation at the cellular level, making it a great option for arthritis sufferers.

- Turmeric, also called curcumin, is known as a great anti-inflammatory agent and has been shown to be highly effective, particularly for people managing rheumatoid arthritis (RA). Turmeric acts on a chemical called interleukin (IL)-6, which causes the inflammation specific to RA. Patients take turmeric veggie caps and drink turmeric tea and smoothies.

- Frankincense is a very old oil. It's so old that it is mentioned in the Old Testament. Researchers know that it inhibits the body's production of key inflammatory molecules specific to conditions like arthritis. Frankincense can also help prevent the breakdown of cartilage tissue in the joints, the main cause of arthritis pain. It's truly a natural treatment option for pain-related conditions of the muscles, joints and tendons.

- Myrrh oil is another ancient oil like frankincense. It also has anti-inflammatory properties, and is often used together with frankincense to treat arthritis. Together, the oils suppress the intensity of inflammation in the joints.

- Orange oil also has strong anti-inflammatory properties. Orange oil had the highest level of antioxidants, which makes it a great essential oil for arthritis treatment. Use avocado or almond oil as a carrier oil, then rub into joints wherever you have pain.

Inflammation

More people than ever are suffering from rampant inflammation, which wreaks havoc on so many body systems. Over time, chronic inflammation has drastic effects. The human body is supposed to naturally regulate inflammation, but immune systems are so under fire from stress, pollutants and other factors that many people have inflammation that is out of control. Certain oils like thyme and oregano have a compound called carvacrol that supports the immune system. A group of scientists in 2015 found that carvacrol kept the body from overproducing the inflammatory molecules that lead to negative effects.

Visible inflammation causes pain, redness, immobility, swelling and heat. Yet there are many types of chronic inflammation inside the body which we cannot see. Here are the best oils to help you fight inflammation.

- Peppermint is great for reducing the acute inflammation caused by injury, and can be even more effective when used with lavender and German chamomile in an anti-inflammatory blend.

- Eucalyptus works well on respiratory inflammation--bronchitis, laryngitis, pneumonia. It packs a punch as an anti-inflammatory, antibacterial, decongestant and mucolytic (breaks up mucus). It works well with spruce and spike lavender in a respiratory essential oil blend.

- And speaking of lavender, it also is effective on respiratory inflammation, but also works well in infections and acute inflammation due to injury.

- German chamomile is particularly effective for inflammatory skin conditions

- Spruce oil eases the pain in arthritis or swollen joints. It has analgesic and anti-inflammatory properties.

Healing

Several oils fit the bill to promote general healing:

- Arnica Oil: arnica has long been added to natural pain reliever products. It has natural anti-inflammatory properties and has been shown in research studies to be useful in treating osteoarthritis as well as carpal tunnel syndrome. It's great for acute sports-related injuries.

- Basil oil can really help if you are fighting a cold or allergies. The oil is high in antioxidants and has both antibacterial and antifungal properties. People use it to treat everything from ear infections to urinary tract infections.

- Tea tree oil does so many things. It is extremely versatile and a must-have for any medicine cabinet. It is useful for bacterial infections, insect bites, cold sores, earaches, and even psoriasis. It has tremendous antimicrobial.

- Lavender can induce sleep, which is very important for healing. It is easily the most popular essential oil for its many uses. Lavender can be helpful in diabetes management because it balances blood sugar.

- Peppermint oil is really effective against several types of digestive disorders, like indigestion or irritable bowel syndrome.

-

Energy Boost

Who doesn't need an energy boost, practically daily? Here are a few oils you may not realize can give you that much-needed energy boost.

- Basil: There are two types of basil essential oil, exotic basil and French (sweet) basil. French basil is the only one safe to use in aromatherapy; besides, it smells better. Basil oil is known to stimulate the adrenal glands, releasing hormones that help fight mental fatigue. Basil is often blended with lime, spearmint and rosemary.

- Ginger essential oil has an invigorating effect on nerves, and can pep you up even if you got no sleep. It is often blended with lime essential oil.

- Speaking of lime, this essential oil is a great restorative. Use it if you've had trouble concentrating. It blends well with basil, ginger, and rosemary.

- Mint oils like peppermint and spearmint do act similarly. Spearmint is the milder of the two. It can have a tremendous calming effect on the nervous system.

- Rosemary essential oil is a stimulant, and can give you that boost you sorely need. People use it when mental fatigue or low energy set in.

Digestion

More and more, we're learning that a healthy digestive system is foundational to good health. Many Americans have gut issues and are looking for a natural way to restore their gastrointestinal comfort and normal digestion. Look no further than essential oils:

Peppermint has long been associated with soothing stomach aches and providing gastrointestinal comfort. It supports healthy gut bacteria and makes digestion more efficient.

Pregnancy and childbirth

For thousands of years, midwives have used essential oils to ease the pain of pregnancy and delivery. Modern midwives still use these oils for massage, and patients report less anxiety and pain.

Always check with your midwife or doctor before you use oils during pregnancy. Many oils affect hormone levels and alter your body's functions. For example, peppermint oil is known to decrease milk supply in nursing mothers. Clary sage should only be used by a midwife during labor.

Here are some other oils to avoid while pregnant and nursing: *aniseed, angelica, basil, birch, black pepper, camphor, cinnamon, chamomile, clary sage, clove, cypress, fennel, fir, ginger, hyssop, jasmine, juniper, marjoram, myrrh, nutmeg, oak moss, oregano, parsley seed, pennyroyal, peppermint, rose, rosemary, rue, sage, tarragon, thyme, wintergreen and wormwood.*

The following oils are generally safe during pregnancy, used according to proper dilution methods: *benzoin, bergamot, black pepper, chamomile (German & Roman), clary sage, cypress, eucalyptus, frankincense, geranium, ginger, grapefruit, juniper, lavender, lemon, mandarin, majoram (sweet), neroli, petitgrain, rose, sandalwood, orange (sweet), tea tree, ylang ylang.*

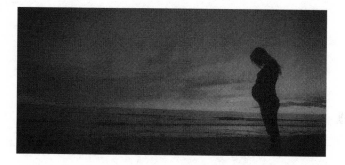

Buying Guide

It is really important to have proper knowledge about buying essential oils. They typically come in 5ml, 10ml and 15ml bottles. Some of the rarer and more expensive oils might be sold in 1ml and 2ml sizes.

The U.S. FDA does not regulate essential oils, so finding a quality distributor is imperative.

Not all essential oils are created equal. There are many worthless products on the market. You'll find many synthetic products, too.

There are four things you want to look for:

- USDA organic certification
- 100 percent pure labeling
- Therapeutic grade oils
- Indigenously sourced oils
- Labeling regarding whether the oil has been diluted

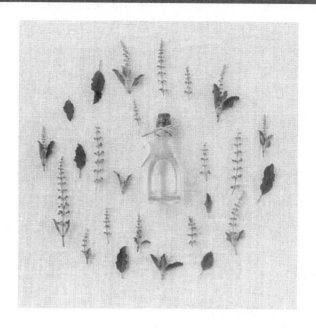

For starters, comparison shop for several brands of the same oil. Most likely the really inexpensive ones are probably diluted, synthetic or made with cheaper ingredients, and not worth your money. Low prices are red flags, unless the company is offering a promotional discount.

Legitimate sellers are transparent about describing their products. Their websites should have quality control documents you can download about the contents of their oils and how they make their product.

Look at the ingredients. Legitimate sellers should list all the ingredients.

Therapeutic grade oils are the highest grade. Wellness grade oils are the next grade and indicate a steam-distilled product; the source plants may have been sprayed with pesticides. Just because an oil says "pure", doesn't mean it is quality. This is the most common form of labeling and the most commonly sold essential oil; normally the oils are over-processed. The lowest grade consists of synthetic and altered oils that have been created in a lab.

Always buy therapeutic grade oils. They're made of the highest quality plants and grown in organic soil. They've been made by steam distillation or cold-pressing without the use of chemicals.

The cost of an essential oil is determined by several factors, including the plant used, the method of production, and the quantity of oil to be produced.

Citrus oils are reasonably affordable whereas rose, jasmine and sandalwood are very costly.

There are subtypes of essential oil, all referred to under the blanket term "essential oil" because they're all natural, concentrated, liquid aromatics, just obtained by different methods.

- Absolutes: made from rare botanicals like jasmine and rose, solvent extraction is used to obtain the precious oil.

- CO2 Extracts: CO2-extracted oils use carbon dioxide as a solvent. The CO_2 is converted to liquid under low temperature, high pressure conditions. The active components and oils of the plant are then collected in the cool liquid. When extraction is complete, the carbon dioxide is reverted to its gaseous form. Left behind are the essential oils.

It is important to remember that essential oils and fragrance oils are definitely not the same things. Essential oils are the true aromatic essence of the plant and are highly concentrated. Furthermore, essential oils are usually not referred to as fragrances.

Fragrance oils are usually listed as just "fragrance" in an ingredient list. These oils are generally synthetic and therefore much less expensive than essential oils.

Typically available in hundreds of scents, many products can be created with fragrance oils that mimic natural essential oils scents.

Because they're synthetic, fragrance oils are much more likely to cause allergies or skin irritation in individuals who use them. This is the very reason why many people opt for perfume-free products like laundry detergent and lotions. Essential oils are considered much less gentle.

Just because a product contains a fragrance oil doesn't mean it is of inferior quality. Its use is often a trade-off in cost. When manufacturers make candles or soaps, it takes a lot more essential oil to create the fragrance. That is why many products are all natural, such as beeswax candles or soap, except for the fragrance.

To tell the difference, just know that products with fragrance oils are not allowed to be listed as being 100% natural, because they're not. The fragrances are synthetic. A fragrance oil may be listed as "lavender fragrance" while an essential oil containing product will be listed as *Lavandula officinalis* (lavender oil).

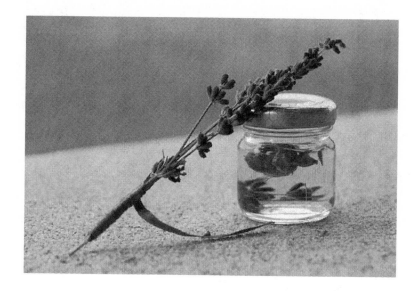

How to store essential oils

Most essential oils come in dark glass containers to keep light out since light and UV rays can change the oils by creating oxidation. Store oils in a cool place. Once opened, most oils can be safely used for one to two years.

Essential oils typically do not become rancid, but they do oxidize and therefore lose their beneficial properties. Citrus oils are particularly susceptible to oxidation, sometimes losing their effectiveness in as little as six months.

Other oils mature with age, like patchouli and sandalwood.

Properly store oils in dark brown or blue bottles; these dark glasses shield the oils from sunlight, which can deteriorate the oils. It's the same reason why most bottled beers are stored in brown bottles. It is unwise to store your oils in clear bottles or plastic bottles. Some oils will degrade the plastic and ruin the oil in a short amount of time.

Some vendors sell oils in aluminum bottles, which is fine as long as the bottles are lined so the oil does not interact with the metal.

Also try not to purchase essential oils with a rubber dropper as a cap. Always buy oils with a screw top cap. The dropper should be separate as the oil will degrade the rubber. Rather than a dropper bottle, it is acceptable to purchase small bottles with a top called an orifice reducer, which is a small, clear insert that fits inside the bottle to serve as a built-in dropper. To use it, tip the bottle to dispense the oil drops. The reducers are made of materials that stand up to any oil. If your oils come with the orifice reducers, it is one indication that you are purchasing a high-quality oil.

Always store oils in a cool, dark place, such as a wooden box with a lid. Better yet, refrigerate your oils if possible.

Essential Oil Starter Kit

If you could purchase just 10 well-rounded oils, what would they be? Here is a suggestion of a top 10 list.

- Bergamot's citrusy aroma is great for healing skin and lifting moods

- Clove oil is perfect for pain relief and inflammation and great for inflamed gum tissues

- Eucalyptus oil is a great decongestant and topical pain reliever

- Frankincense has anti-microbial and anti-inflammatory properties and is one of the oldest oils in the world

- Lavender is calming and sleep-inducing

- Lemon oil is anti-fungal and an all-around household cleaner and air freshener

- Oregano helps skin conditions like eczema and psoriasis

- Peppermint aids digestion and eases headaches

- Rosemary detoxifies and helps skin and hair, and you can cook with it!

- Tea tree (melaleuca) helps skin and scalp

The Best Oils To Have In Your Medicine Cabinet

What if you could build a medicine cabinet just out of essential oils? What would you choose? You'd need headache relief, insect sting remedies and sunburn relief. Here is a recommendation for a natural essential oil medicine cabinet without the side effects of conventional drugs like aspirin and antibiotics.

- Lavender for cuts, stings, burns, and rashes. It also reduces anxiety and helps you fall asleep.
- Peppermint helps headaches and muscle and joint pain. It also helps with digestive issues and asthma and bronchitis. This wonder oil can also reduce fever and clear sinuses.
- Frankincense is a powerful anti-inflammatory agent with all sorts of uses.
- Melaleuca (tea tree) is both an antibacterial and antifungal. It can reduce or even prevent infection and can clean the air of allergens.

- You may want to also have some eucalyptus, oregano and clove on hand. Oregano acts like an antibiotic, and the others have multiple remedies.

Essential Oils for Weight Loss

You may have heard about people using essential oils for weight loss, and there are some oils that can help. Keep in mind that the oils just help with weight loss. They are not a cure all. Dietary changes and exercise are the mainstays, but oils can provide an extra boost to help you reach a weight loss goal. The oils are much more natural than caffeine and other stimulants. These four oils help support fat loss:

- Peppermint oil suppresses cravings and improves digestion
- Grapefruit oil contains the compound d-limonene found in citrus peels. D-limonene improves metabolic enzyme levels which speeds up your metabolism.
- Cinnamon bark oil helps to balance blood sugar levels. When those levels are balanced, weight loss is easier.
- Ginger oil contains gingerol, which decreases inflammation and increases thermogenesis, turning each cell into a fat burning factory that boosts metabolism.

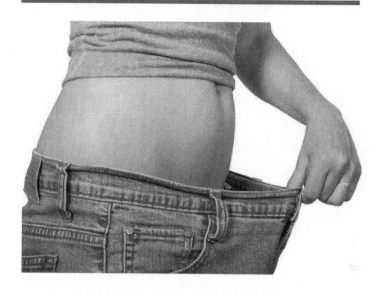

Best Essential Oil Remedies

When you look at this long list of remedies, it is clear to see that essential oils have some incredible properties.

- Migraine headache relief
- Reduce cough or sinus pressure
- Heal burns
- Soothe bug bites
- Improve digestion
- Bronchitis and asthma remedy
- Treat bruises
- Improve concentration

- Sore feet soak

- Reduce teeth grinding

- Relieve PMS

- Eczema and psoriasis cream

- Improve circulation

- Relieve hangover symptoms

- Curb food cravings

- Energize your workout

- Reduce fever

- Relieve motion sickness

- Arthritis relief

- Treat ringworm

- Head lice treatment

- Heal blistered skin

- Soothe a sunburn

- Treat poison oak

- Lose weight

- Boost immune system

- Sore muscles

- Reduce morning sickness

- Improve allergies

- Kick a cold

- Reduce back and neck pain

Home Uses

Essential oils can be used throughout the home to support wellness through a clean environment.

- First, lemon is a powerful all-purpose cleaner that leaves a fresh, clean scent. It is a natural disinfectant. Add a few drops of tea tree for an added boost.

- Spray your kids sports gear with a mixture of the lemon/tea tree with four tablespoons of baking soda added to warm water. It will definitely disinfect and de-funkify those ripe-smelling uniforms and shoes.

- Cinnamon is a natural anti-microbial that is great sprayed in the air.

- Add 20 drops of your favorite oil to every laundry load, and it will not only make those clothes and sheets smell great, it will keep your washing machine smelling great too.

- Add some drops of any oil to your vacuum cleaner and it won't smell dusty any more.

- You can make your own sunscreen from essential oils. Just mix coconut oil with some zinc oxide and shea butter, then add lavender and helichrysum oils. Mix together and store in a squeeze bottle. You'll be sun free and toxin free too.

- Every home has had yucky shower curtain scum from time to time. Fill a spray bottle with warm water and add four drops each of eucalyptus and tea tree essential oils and you'll have a natural mold-killer that will get rid of the scum. Add tea tree oil to your diffuser to kill mold and other pathogens in the air.

- Who hasn't experienced a burnt-bottom kitchen pan at one time or another? Never fear. Just add some water and lemon oil and boil.

- Have a great smelling home by diffusing a blend of orange, clove and rosemary. Your house will smell amazing. Guests will comment.

- You can make your own homemade carpet freshening powder out of borax and 20 drops of tea tree oil.

- Don't use harsh pesticides. Make a mixture of orange and clove oils and spray your pest. It will be killed on contact.

- Add a couple of drops of lemon oil to a bowl of water and wash all your fruit and vegetables

- A clove, cinnamon and citrus essential oil mixture in a simmering pan of water will get rid of cooking odors

- Combine a half cup each of vinegar and baking soda with bergamot or lime oil and use it to scrub your sink or tub.

- To freshen your trash can place a cotton ball soaked in lemon oil to cut down of trash odor.

You can do the same and place a cotton ball behind your toilet.

- Rinse your refrigerator with a water mixture containing lime, grapefruit or bergamot oil

- Make a blend of eucalyptus, tea tree and rosemary oils to eliminate cigar or cigarette smoke from your home.

- Add lemon oil to your dishwasher. You'll have cleaner spot-free dishes and a great smelling dishwasher

Industrial Uses

Essential oils have long been used in industrial cleaning products. If you smell that lemon furniture polish or that almond-scented floor cleaner, chances are it contains an essential oil. Many pest control products contain oils like citronella. Vicks Vaporub has eucalyptus oil.

Hospital Use

Hospitals are using oils for aromatherapy and to reduce infections. Vanderbilt University Hospital, for example, regularly uses the oils to treat depression and anxiety, but also to reduce infections.

Research studies show that patients who did lavender aromatherapy prior to surgery were less anxious about it.

Midwives also use specific essential oils to reduce fear and anxiety during labor. Essential oils can also have antibacterial or antifungal benefits and can be used to keep equipment clean.

Hospitals are definitely catching on to essential oils, using them to treat burns, as a sleep aid, for massage and to boost the immune system.

There are even studies underway to determine whether certain essential oils like frankincense can help fight cancer.

Veterinary Uses

Essential oils can absolutely be used in veterinary applications on animals. In fact, the use of synthetic repellents for fleas and other pests is becoming very problematic. Animals, like humans, develop sensitivities or allergic reactions. A blend of citronella, lemon and eucalyptus essential oils has been used with success, and citronella, clove and lily of the valley oils have been effective against ticks—just as effective in fact as the chemical DEET, but without all the toxic side effects.

Dogs and cats suffer from several fungal skin conditions that cause excessive itching. A blend of essential oils (lavender, bitter orange, oregano, marjoram, peppermint and helichrysum) with carriers, coconut oil and sweet almond oil, proved effective. In the study, animals treated for one month with the oil blend fared the same as the medicated control group.

Tea tree oil has been used effectively to fight mites. Tea tree oil is very toxic to pets unless used in the right concentrations by a trained veterinarian. The Journal of the American Veterinary Association reported hundreds of incidents of tea tree oil toxicity in pets in a 10 year period. Dogs and cats cannot tolerate pure tea tree oil in the same concentration that a human can.

In the same way, aromatherapy may have adverse effects on your pets for the same reasons. Larger animals tolerate it well. In fact, there have even been research studies showing lavender's effectiveness on horses by keeping them calm.

Veterinarians on commercial farms are also putting essential oils into practice. Many farmers are adding the oils to food to keep their intestinal health strong and to fight infections. Farmers who are raising antibiotic-free poultry say that they regularly use oregano oil and cinnamon oil to fight infection on farms. It has an amazing effect on gut bacteria in the animals. The oregano oil kills the bad bacteria and cinnamon oil supports the good bacteria.

Culinary Uses

Food is central to all world cultures. It's always present in times of celebration. So many people around the world love to cook; great cooks are always looking for new herbs, spices and flavor combinations.

Have you ever thought about cooking with essential oils? Lots of great cooks do. In fact, you likely already do, too, without realizing it. Every time you add olive oil or avocado oil to a dish, you're cooking with essential oils.

However, you may not have tried oils as flavoring agents, but you should. You'll be surprised at how the addition of one or two drops of oil adds flare to a recipe. Just remember that there is a significant

So, the idea that cooking with essential oils or incorporating them into our kitchen process is nothing new. The important thing is to do it safely, appreciating the differences between a whole herb or spice and its essential oil.

You'll also want to note that not every essential oil is a good choice for cooking. Sometimes cooking with essential oils doesn't taste quite as yummy as the whole herb.

Cooking with essential oils is pretty easy and it adds so much flavor to food. How great would it be to just add two drops of oil instead of all that chopping?

Because essential oil is so concentrated, you're using a much smaller portion when you cook. There's not a one-size-fits-all rule for how to convert whole herbs to oil, but in general, one drop of oil is equal to one teaspoon of chopped fresh or dried herbs or spices.

When you cook with an oil, you're going to use a similar carrier oil concept. Always dilute your drops of essential oil into a fat—olive oil, coconut oil, chicken fat, butter—whatever your recipe calls for. The fat helps disperse the oil into the entire dish so it's not just concentrated in one area.

If you're making a dessert, you can disperse the oil into syrup or honey. If you're creating a hot dish, add the essential oil at the very end of the cooking process. Remember they're volatile and they'll burn off easily, especially under high heat. Most cooks remove the dish from the heat, then stir in the diluted oil.

Cooks are sometimes hesitant to use essential oils because they feel that the heat damages the oil's properties, in particular by evaporation or alteration of the oil's chemical structures. It can happen, but the best way to prevent it is to minimize heat exposure.

Just remember that when you cook with essential oils, it's not so much that you're using the oil for health benefits. Rather, you're adding the oil for flavor and aroma of the dish.

Here are 10 staple oils you should have in your kitchen:

- Lavender is a very gentle oil with a delicate flavor for desserts and fish. You can even flavor lemonade with it.
- Peppermint is cool and refreshing in tea, lemonade and lots of desserts, especially chocolate ones.
- Citrus oils are great for cooking and you can use them in almost anything from smoothies to stir-fry.
- Bergamot is a citrus, but it is different. It's not a fruit that is normally eaten so its oil essence is a special treat in tea and scones.
- Cinnamon is most known for cookie flavoring, but it excellent in any sweet dish.
- Cardamom pairs well with cinnamon and is the flavor you taste when you drink chai. Cardamom can be used in any dessert that calls for spices and is also good on meat.
- Ginger root is used in gingerbread, stir fry and lots of marinades.

- Thyme is a favorite culinary herb that is good in meat dishes, soups and stews. It's excellent on poultry.
- Anise is famous for its licorice flavor, and can be added to any kind of cookie, but is great in marinades and soups too. Anise has a similar flavor to fennel and is good on meat, chicken or fish.
- Coriander/cilantro are from the same plant. Coriander is the seed and cilantro is the leaf. Their flavors are drastically different. Cilantro oil can be added to salsas, while coriander oil goes great in savory dishes, sauces and vegetable dishes.

What Does Research Say?

Even though essential oils have been used for medical remedies for thousands of years, there is still very little published research on the topic. But that is beginning to change, as the potential power of essential oils is becoming more evident. Studies are going on around the world, in countries like Europe, Australia, Japan, India, the United States, and Canada.

The research is certainly being done by industries, like the food and cosmetics industries, but also by agricultural outlets looking for a non-antibiotic way to raise livestock. They're looking at flavoring that can be provided by essential oils, but also looking at its food preservative qualities as well as adding it to livestock food. Some companies are conducting extensive research on toxicity and safety.

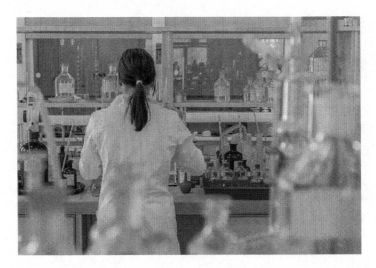

Since it is corporate research, much of it is under wraps, but it is starting to make its way into scientific journals. Results are promising. It is important for scientists to keep adding to journals to grow our body of knowledge on essential oils. It's important to say that many studies to date have been animal studies and have not been conducted on humans, but that is taking shape as the research progresses.

Here are some of the issues that researchers have pointed out.

- Essential oils are not standardized. Plant chemistry is affected by local growing conditions and weather, as well as harvest time and season. As such, no two oils are exactly the same, unlike pharmaceutical drugs that are reproduced to be identical. If you alter an essential oil to make it standard, then it is no longer natural.

- There are not enough blind studies. The oils are so fragrant, you can't hide what you're studying. People associate smells with past experiences, so these studies are difficult to execute.

- There is not much funding of essential oil research. There are not many who want to sponsor research that doesn't follow a conventional clinical research approach of testing in the lab, then animals then humans. Most researchers want to jump straight to testing on humans because of oils' long history and known safety. The pharmaceutical industry funds most of these studies; they're not motivated to fund research that will directly compete with their conventional products.

- It is difficult to determine the study outcome. For example, oils are used in massage. Was the outcome due solely to the oil, to the massage or to both? Furthermore, essential oils are composed of hundreds of chemicals and it is hard to determine the active one or ones.

Despite these concerns, research does appear promising, and shows positive effects in a whole host of areas, including infections, pain, anxiety, depression, tumors, premenstrual syndrome and nausea.

In closing, let's dispel the most common myths about essential oils. It's important to separate fact from fiction for a clear picture of the benefits of these oils going forward.

Myth: Specific oils are the only ways to treat certain conditions.

There is no "one oil, one ailment" mantra. Certainly you must keep the ailment or condition in mind, but there are multiple oil solutions to a particular issue. Always remember--there are many paths to wellness.

Myth: You should take essential oils every day for disease prevention.

You don't take something every day in case you get a toothache, so you likely don't need to take essential oils every day unless you need something. Good holistic practices will get you pretty far in life. Taking or inhaling a certain oil every day won't guarantee you won't get sick, but they will certainly help.

Myth: Essential oils can't be used on pets.

Many vets are treating pets with essential oils. Just know that certain oils might be toxic because pets will not tolerate the oils as humans do. Talk to your vet about using aromatherapy around pets to determine its safety. In particular, cats might be susceptible to essential oils because they lack a liver enzyme that other animals have, therefore substances might be more toxic to cats because they can't process it.

Myth: Essential oils must always be blended and can only be used topically.

Both of these are false. Oils can be used topically, in aromatherapy and even ingested. They do not always have to be diluted for use either. Some can be used full strength.

Myth: Essential oils expire

Essential oils don't expire. If not stored in brown bottles, they can be affected by light exposure which can limit their shelf life. Some age well over time. Many people use expired therapeutic oils for cleaning applications.

Myth: Essential oils are only useful for therapeutic reasons.

Absolutely false. As you've read in this book, oils are used for a variety of important functions on our planet.

Aromatherapy is definitely in the mainstream as a healing art, and it's good to be recognized in that way, but essential oils have many applications, including culinary, agricultural and industrial. The sky is the limit as researchers and companies unlock the great potential of essential oils.

Summary

Although oils like frankincense have been used for thousands of years, we are on the cusp of the next great research revelation in finding out about more essential oils and the positive effects they have on the human body. The near future will be an exciting new era as researchers embark upon this journey to determine what essential oils truly are, and more importantly, what they're not.

If you enjoyed learning about essential oils from this guide, I would be forever grateful if you could leave a review on Amazon. Reviews are by far the best way to help newer authors, like myself, out. It also helps your fellow readers sort through and find the good books so make sure to help them out. Thanks so much in advance for your review!